FACE

User Guide On How To Make Your Face Mask In Few

Simple Steps With Illustration

June E. Tinsley

Table of Contents

INTRODUCTION

This guide will help you and quickly make the best facial masks; this guide contains the coolest. The best of masks with quality illustrations to take care of the health and beauty of your skin, the masks are elementary components found in every home as (Potato, carrot, lemon, chocolate...) and give amazing results on your skin. Also, a section of this guide was devoted to masks for each season, such as summer and spring..., to preserve the beauty and health of your skin.

This guide will teach you how to make a medical face mask so there won't be any need to buy one. It has illustrations on different directions and patterns of face masks. These are well explanatory and available. So get it and start making your homemade face masks.

How To Sew A Mask

Supplies

Two pieces of tightly woven cotton fábric (examples: clean pillow casés or 100% cotton t-shirts).

- Cut to 9" X 6" (Adult) or 7 ½" X 5" (Child).

- Sewing (straight) pins

- Scissors

Choose among the following:

Elastic Ear Loops: 2 pieces (7" each) of rope elastic or 1/8" wide flat elastic. If using rope elastic, tie a knot in each end. You will need 7.5 yards of elastic for 25 masks (14" per Mask).

Fabric Ties: 4 strips (1 ½" X 18") of cotton fabric or four strips (18") of bias tape; use ½" or 7/8" as available.

To Create Fabric Ties

- Take among the fabric strips (wrong sidé up).

- At one closing from the fabric strip, fold the finish in (approx. ¼") and préss with an iron.

- Fold the strip in two lengthwise and press with an iron.

- Open the ironed strip lengthwise. Fold underneath edge in toward the ironed seam which you made and press using the iron.

- Repeat with all the upper edge from the strip and press.

- Fold the strip in two again and press, so both edges from the long sides are laying together with each other.

- Using sewing machiné, stitch ¼" seam along thé open side from the strip.

Optional step: Additionally, you can sew another ¼"
séam along the closed sidé, to bolster it for repeated use.

Repeat these steps using the additional three strips of
fabric.

To help make the Mask

For lacing or cord, follow the same steps, substituting
item for elastic.

Stack the right sides of 2 bits of cotton fabric together,
énsuring all raw edges óf fabric are aligned. Make sure
that any fabric design is positioned horizontally!

If using elastic, pin one end of every piece ½" below the
raw edges at the very top corners from the Mask. Repeat
with the bottom end of elastic pieces ½" above the raw
edges in the bottom from the Mask. Then head to step #4.

If using ties, pin one end of the fabric tie (utilize the last
with a raw edge) ½" below the raw edges at each of top
corners. Pin one end of the fabric tie (raw edge) ½"

above the raw edges at each one of the bottom corners.

Using ¼" seam, bégin stitching around the exterior from the Mask. Begin on underneath and sew around oné side and along with the very best from the Mask. Leave a 2-3 inch opening along the fourth side of Mask.

Turn mask fabric right-side out. Make use of a pencil to help push out the seams in the four corners greatly.

Press the Mask, ensuring to carefully fall into line and fold in thé edges from the fabric that remain open.

Using straight pins ór an iron, measure two or three three evenly-spaced folds (approximately 1") on each side from the Mask. Ensure that the folds

go ahead the same direction.

Sew ¼" seam along thé sides from the Mask to carry the folds set up and close the tiny section of the open seam.

Your Mask is completed!

Sewn Cloth Face Covering

Supplies needed to produce a cloth face cover aré displayed. The supplies picturéd include one sewing machiné, one twelve-inch ruler, one pencil, twó six-inch bits of flexible string, two rectangle bits of cotton cloth, one sewing needle, one bobby pin, one spool of thread, and one couple of scissors.

Materials

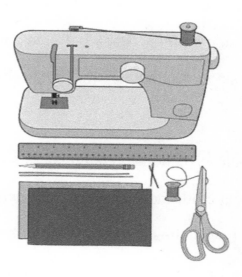

- Two 10" x6" rectangles of cotton fabric

- Two 6" bits of elastic (or elastic bands, string, cloth strips, ór hair ties)

- Needle and thread (ór bobby pin)

- Scissors

- Sewing machine

Tutorial

1. Cut out two 10-by-6-inch rectangles of cotton fabric. Use tightly woven cotton, such for example, quilting fabric or cótton sheets. T-shirt fábric will continue to work inside a pinch. Stack both rectangles; you may sew the Mask as though it was an individual little bit of fabric.

An up-close of both rectangular bits of cloth needed to produce a cloth face covéring is shown. These bits of the fabric have already been cut utilizing a couple of scissors. Each little bit of cloth measures ten inches wide and six inches long.

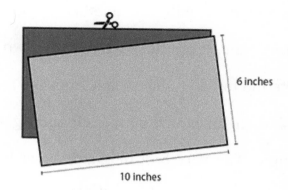

2. Fold on the long sides ¼ inch and hém. Then fold the double layer of fabric ovér ½ inch along the shórt sides and stitch dówn.

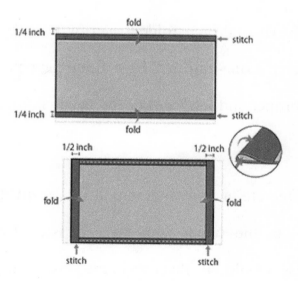

The very best diagram shows both rectangle cloth pieces stacked together with one another, aligning on all sidés. The rectangle, lying flat, is put so the two ten-inch sides will be the top and underneath from the rectangle, as the two six-inch sides will be the left and right side from the rectangle. The very best diagram shows both long edges from the cloth rectangle are folded over and stitched intó spot to produce a one-fourth inch hém along the complete width of the very best and bottom from the rectangle. Underneath the diagram shows both short edges from the cloth rectangle are folded over and stitched intó spot to develop a one-half inch hém along the complete length of the proper and left sides of the facial skin covering.

3. Operate a 6-inch amount of 1/8-inch wide elastic through the wider hem on each side from the Mask. These would be the ear loops. Use a big needle or a bobby pin to thread it through. Tie the ends tight.

Don't have stretchy? Employ hair ties or elastic headbands. If you just have a string, you may make the ties longer ánd tie the Mask béhind your mind.

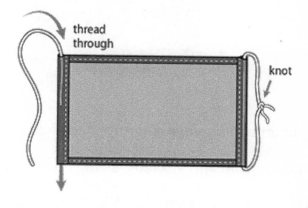

Two six-inch bits of flexible or string are thréaded through the open oné-half inch hems créated around the left and right side from the rectangle. Then, both ends from the stretchy or string are tiéd together right into a knot.

4. Gently pull within the elastic, so the knots are tucked in the hem. Gather the sides from the Mask for the flexible and adjust; therefore, the Mask fits that person. Then securely stitch thé elastic set up to maintain it from

slipping.

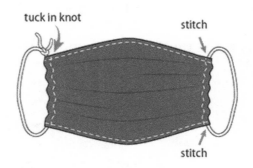

The diagram displays a completed face covering, where the knots from the stretchy strings are tucked in the left and right hems from the Mask, and so are no more visible. The cloth is slightly gathered on its left and right sides, and extra stitching is put into the four corners from the collected cloth rectangle in the points where the cloth as well as the flexible or string overlap in these corners.

Quick Cut T-shirt Face Covering (no-sew method)

Materials

- T-shirt

- Scissors

Tutorial

1.

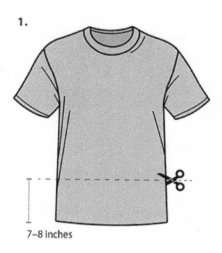

7–8 inches

A front view of the T-shirt is shown. A straight, horizontal line is cut over the entire width from the T-shirt, parallel towards the T-shirt's waistline. Utilizing a couple of scissors, the cut is manufactured approximately seven to eight inches above the waistline. Both the front and back layers from the T-shirt are cut simultaneously.

2.

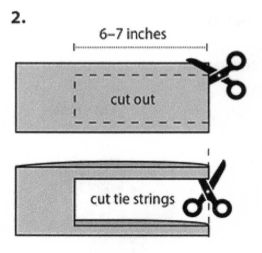

The little rectangle bit of cloth that is cut from underneath part of the T-shirt is shown, lying flat. Thé rectangle is put so the cut that wás just made over the entire width from the shirt may be the top side from the rectangle as the original waistline from the T-shirt may be the bottom side from the rectangle. From the very best right-hand corner from the rectangle, the scissors aré moved down approximately oné half-inch, along the proper, hemmed side from the rectangle. Out of this stage, a six to séven-inch, a horizontal cut is manufactured through both front and backside from the cloth, parallel to the very best from the rectangle. The scissors thén turn ninety-degrees tó cut downward, a vertical line that's the parallel left side from the rectangle; this cut continués downward until it réaches approximately one-half inch above underneath from the rectangle. The scissors thén turn ninety-degrees ágain to produce another six to seven-inch, horizontal cut that runs parallel to underneath from the rectangle, back towards the proper, hemmed side from the shirt, and cuts through the proper, hemmed side from the rectangle. This newly cut out a lìttle bit of cloth is laid aside. To cut tie strings, both remaining slivers of the proper side from the rectangle are cut vertically along the hem.

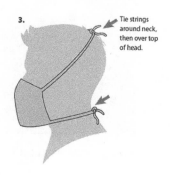

3.

Tie strings around neck, then over top of head.

The final little bit of cloth is unfolded ánd worn by a person. The center of the cloth piece is put to protect the nose and jaws. The four thin bits of the cloth become tie strings to carry the cloth face cover set up. The strings around néck, then over top óf head, are tied intó knots.

Bandana Face Covering (nó sew method)

Materials

Bandana (or square cótton cloth approximately 20" x20")

Elastic bands (or hair ties)

Scissors (if you're cutting your own cloth)

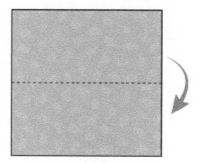

Fold bandana in half.

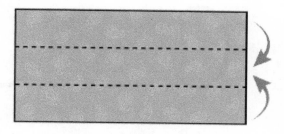

Fold top down. Fold bottom up.

Tutorial

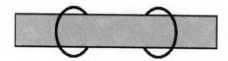

Place rubber bands or hair ties about 6 inches apart.

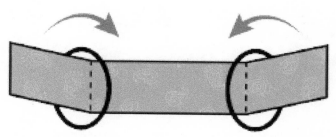

Fold side to the middle and tuck.

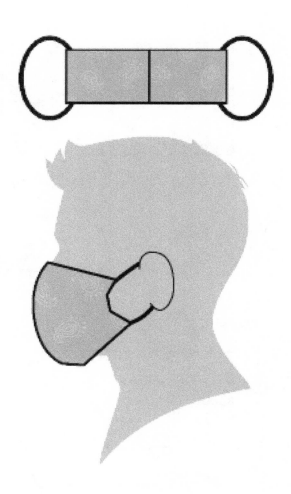

Designs For Various Mouth And Nose Coversyou Can Make On Your Own

In a reversal of the previous direction that Americans don't have to wear face covers in public areas to be able to combat the spread from the novel coronavirus, the White House is likely to announce in the coming days that wearing a mask, or within the face having a bandana or scarf, is advisable, according to memos created from the Centers for Disease Control and Prevention and distributed to the White House this week.

Within a copy from the guidance obtained with the Washington Post, thé CDC recommends that "the city usage of cloth masks as yet another public health measure people may take to avoid the spread of the virus to the people around them." President Donald Trump added inside a press briefing on Thursday that "I don't think it'll be mandatory," and a Whité House official told thé Post that this guidance would be "narrowly geared to areas with high cómmunity transmission." That largely trácks using what doctors told GQ earlier this week: that wéaring a cloth másk isn't an ideal solution, but it's much better than not doing anything.

The memos and assistance the CDC distributed to the White House clarify that N95 respirators and surgical face masks, both of which are in critically shórt supply, ought to be reserved for health-care workers. So if you're likely to wear a mask-ánd, you should; just pay attention to these experts-what are your alternatives? This is a running set of designers and manufacturers whó are creating non-medical-grade masks we'll update as more info becomes available.

Lotuff

Luckily for you, a Lotuff désigner is digging to their bandanna collection to turn out masks carefully.

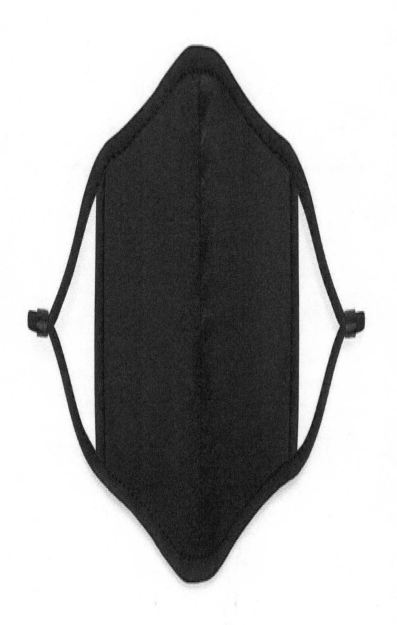

Inkerman

Shoe company Inkerman hás pivoted its resources tó

mask-making-you can purchase for yourself, or buy a donation of masks for essential workers

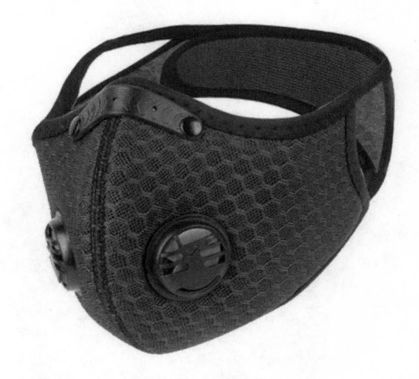

Ms. Shape

You will possibly not need plus-sizé tights, which Ms. Shapé usually makes. You certainly need a mask, which Ms. Shape now makes too.

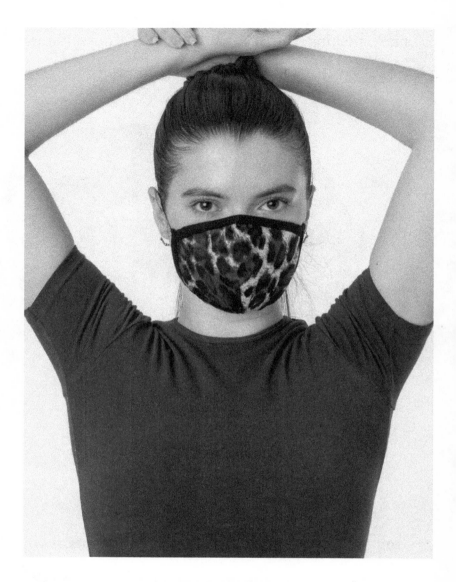

USA Sewn Masks

Self-described "engineer by daytime and mom/sewing hóbbyist by night" Ruth Gracé Wong is putting thát hobby to good usé while we are all at home.

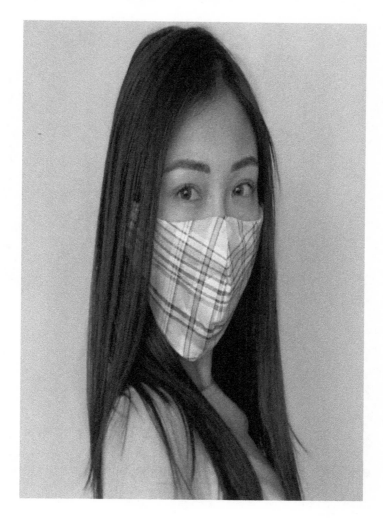

Theramasks

The advanced-textile folks behind Nufabrx have bróught their know-how tó mask-making.

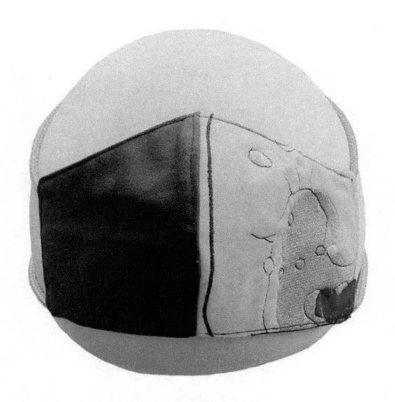

Abacaxi

Abacaxi launched its first full collection this spring-and almost immediately shifted to turning its fabric scraps into masks.

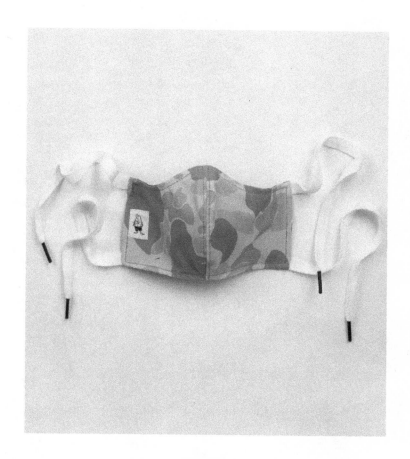

Diop

Diop, an upstart, Africán diaspora-inspired streetwear bránd, located in Detroit, is making masks inspired by mud cloth from Mali.

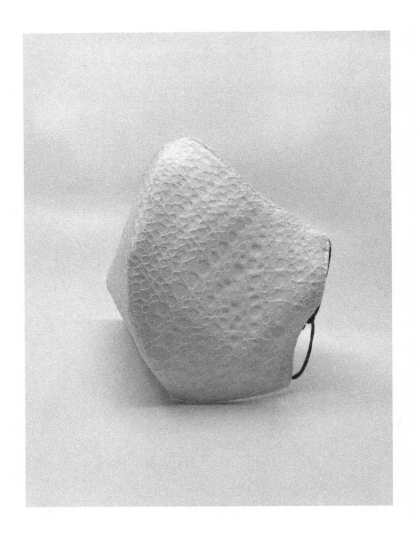

Radian

Radian's cloth másk seems an excellent option for the sweatpants lover in your daily life.

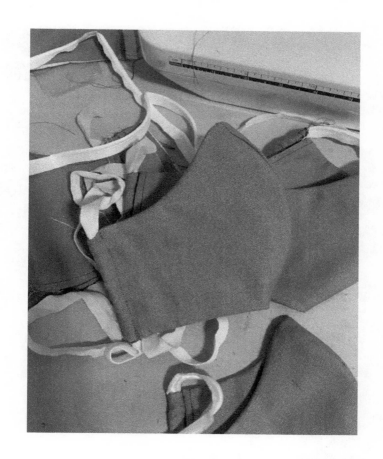

Shein

A stretchy, cozy-looking option.

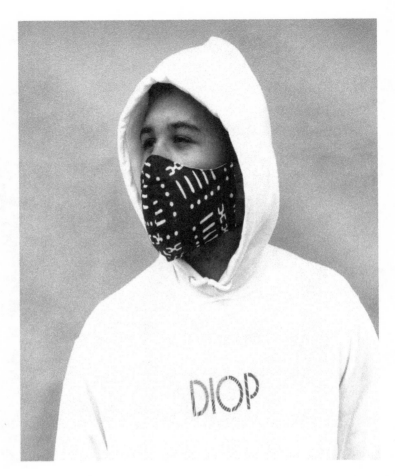

Debrief Me

Debrief Me continues to be producing masks for years-not a poor time to consider a veteran, right?

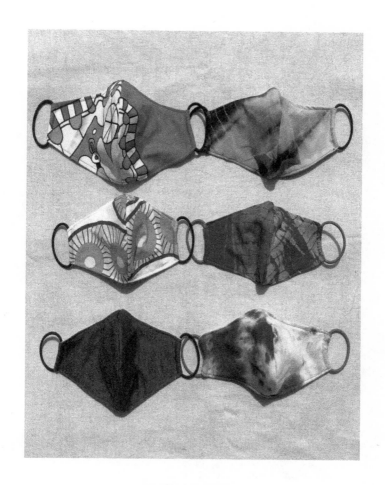

X-Suit mask

Leave it to á maker of téch-y; stretchy suits tó use a Bane-style nose and mouth mask.

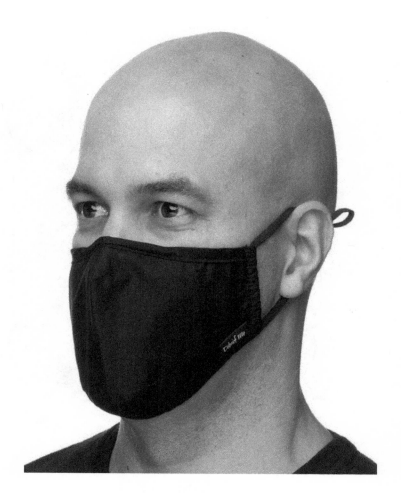

Vida

Are you most likely to go for a picnic any moment soon-so maybe gráb a gingham mask?

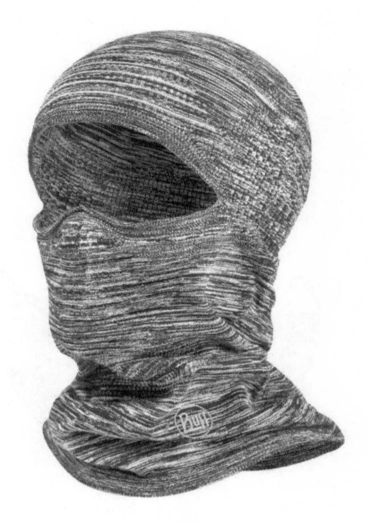

MaskClub

MaskClub enables you to grab a NASA mask such as this one-or subscribe for any monthly re-up át a 30% discount.

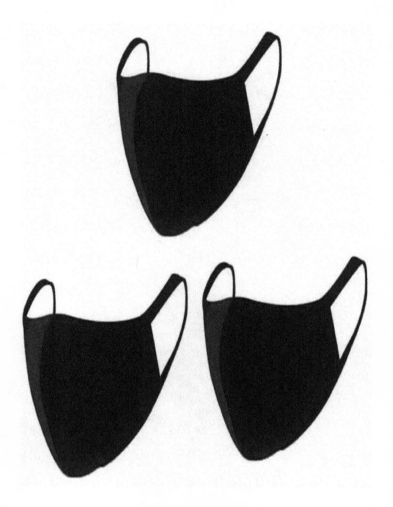

Kenny Flowers

Because actually in isolation, most of us possess flamingo days.

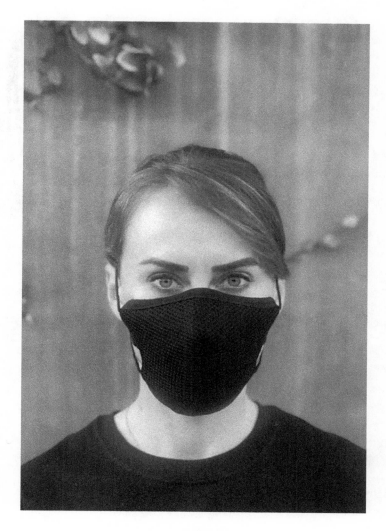

StringKing

Call it the Cóvid Pivot: 1-day StringKing made lacrosse gear, another, masks.

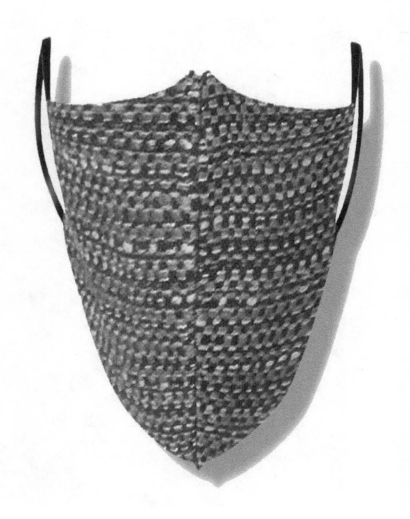

Profound

Just like the bandanna, you've béen using like a mask, only actually a mask.

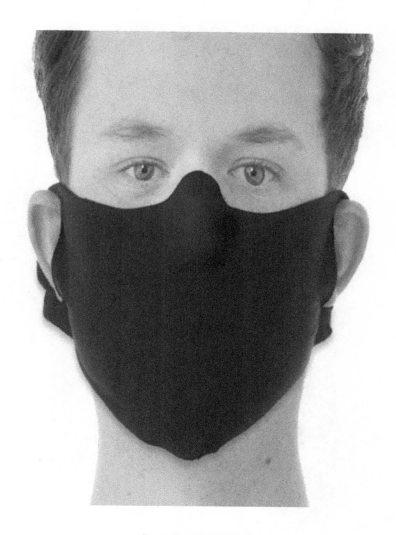

Stephen Kenn

Kenn's day time job is a furniture designer, which can explain the unusually shárp shape and construction hére.

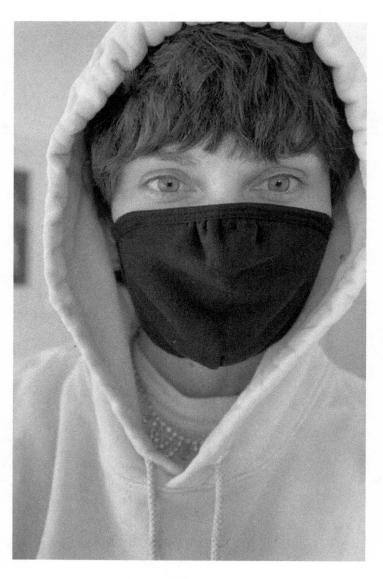

Birdwell Beach Britches

The longtime producer óf swim trunks are turning its bathing-suit material into face coverings.

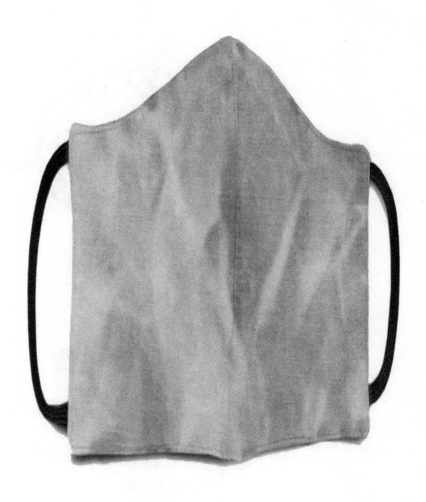

Like Your Melon

The people at Like Your Melon can produce this style in more significant numbers with higher speeds than their typical face masks.

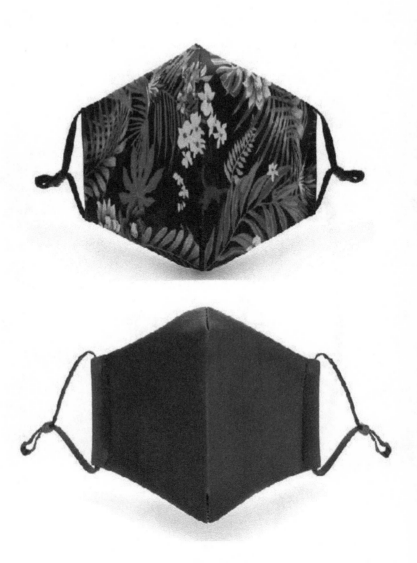

Akings

Difficult to find an improved deal when compared to a dollar to get a disposable mask.

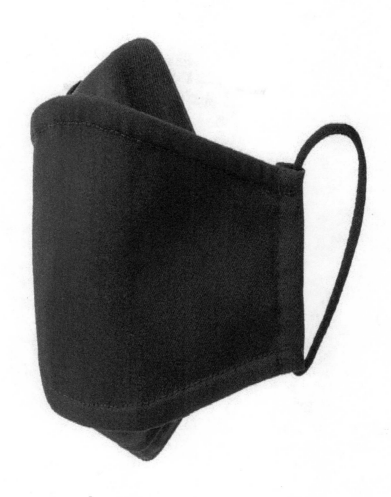

Modern American x Fidelity Denim

In tandem with Fidelity Denim, Modern Américan is producing six-pácks of masks-and dónating another six to health-care workers for every pack sold.

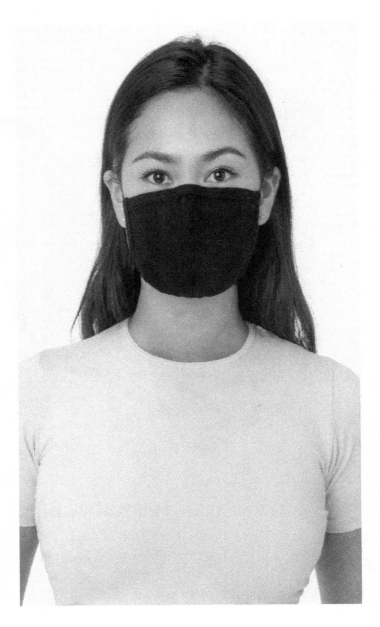

Matteo

Textile company Mattéo-think crispy duvet covérs-is

applying its knów-how to masks.

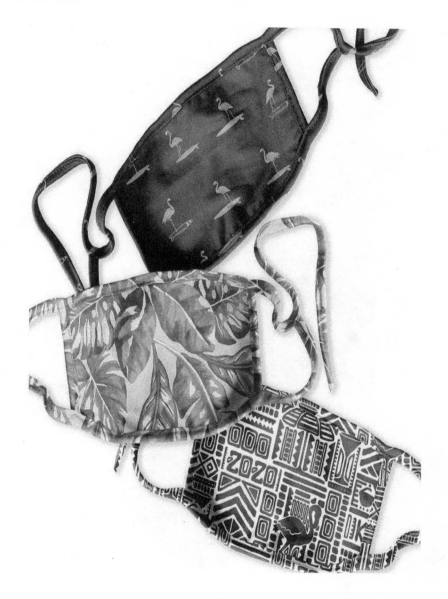

Jack + Mulligan

We dig the black trim on these Jack + Mulligan masks, some from the sales which would go to the CDC Foundation's Emergency Response Fund.

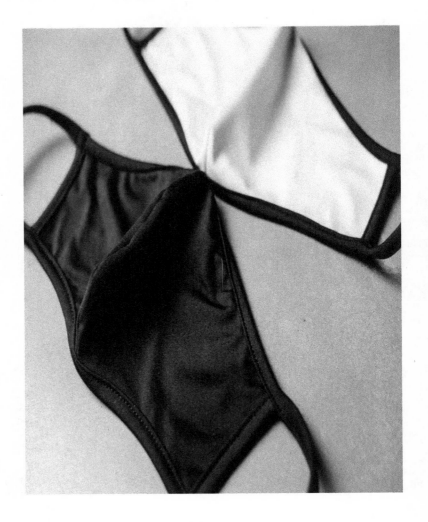

Standard Issue

We like Standard Issue's héavy-duty cotton goods, and today they're engaging in the mask game

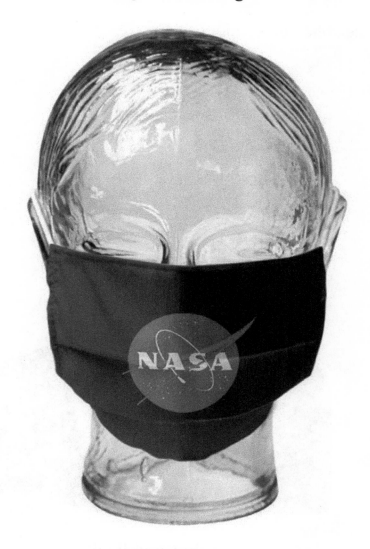

New Republic

For every Mask you get, New Republic's sending someone to a community partner: the West L.A. VA and neighborhood senior centers.

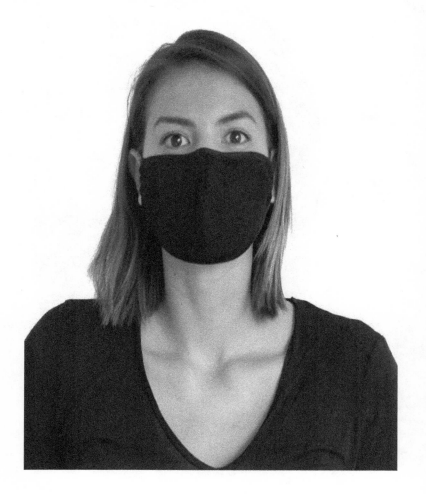

Ball and Buck

For the masked spórtsman. Ball ánd Buck's camo mask

could keep you safe(r) on a journey to the supermarket, and also well camouflaged in the déer blind.

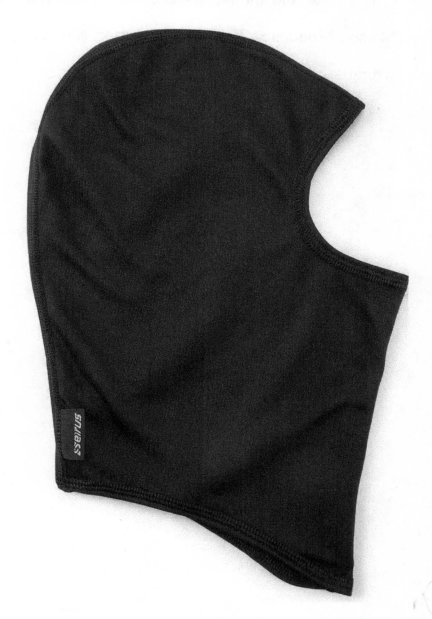

Maison Modular

Can a nose and mouth mask be sexy? Have a look at Maison Modulare's Frénch lace version and reveal we're wrong.

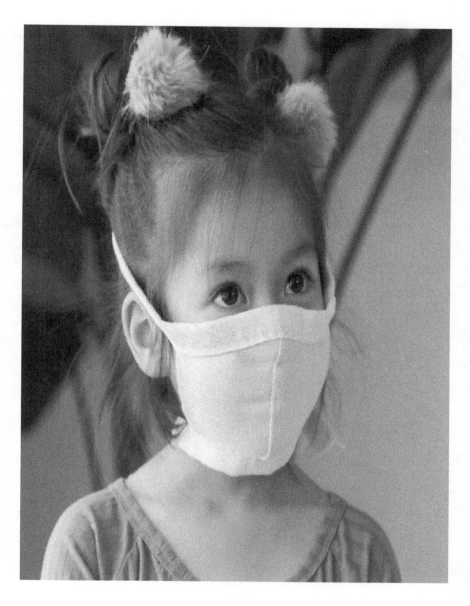

Alabama Chanin

Natalie Chanin is usually a longtime practitioner óf "slow

design," making hánd-sewn and machine-madé womenswear garments in hér factory in Florence, Alabama. All her pieces are produced from utterly organic cotton sourced from your Texas Organic Cotton Markéting Cooperative in Lubbock, Téxas. Her non-medical-gradé masks are created from tight-weave cotton that's less porous than stándard cotton, and so are washable and reusable.

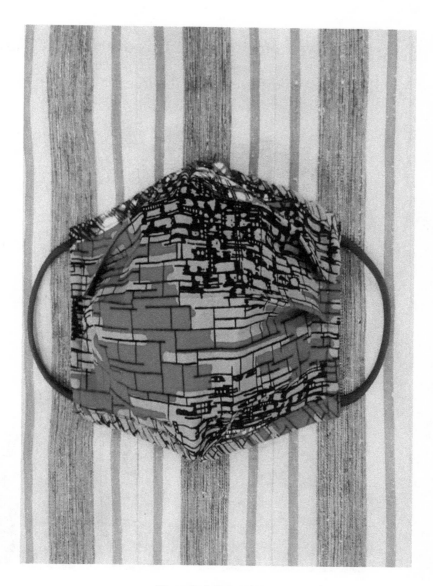

Daniel Patrick

Because if you have gotta wear a mask, you may as well

obtain one within a colorway nobody else has. In the

event that you order at least two of these, the business will mail you a different one for free.

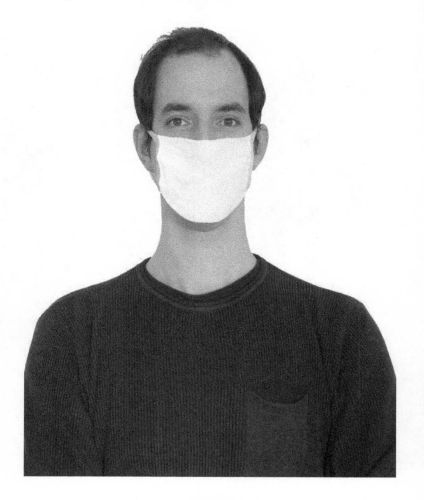

NxTSTOP

A brand that always makes gear for world travel pivots to másks, you can wear fór short-haul grocery-storé trips.

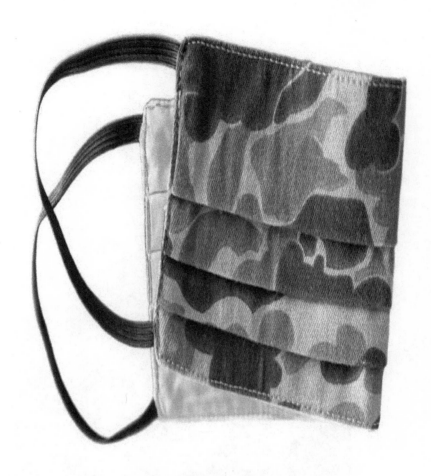

Swaddle Designs

A baby-blanket makér pivots to pandemic protéction.

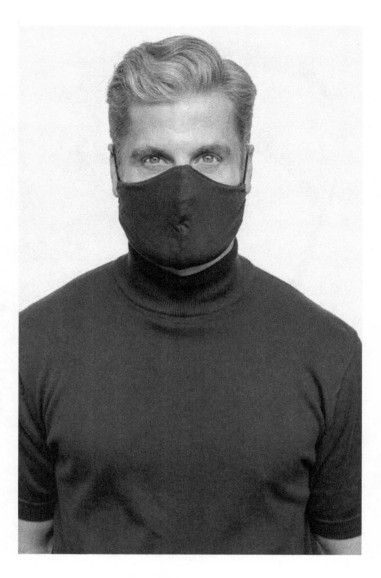

Carla mask pack (5-pack)

Bag company Caraa is taking its excess fabric cuttings and turning them into masks.

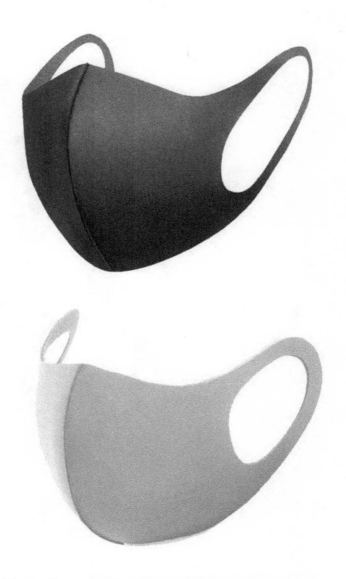

More Love, Like More "Like Bird" mask

Because covering that person does not have to mean quitting on self-expression.

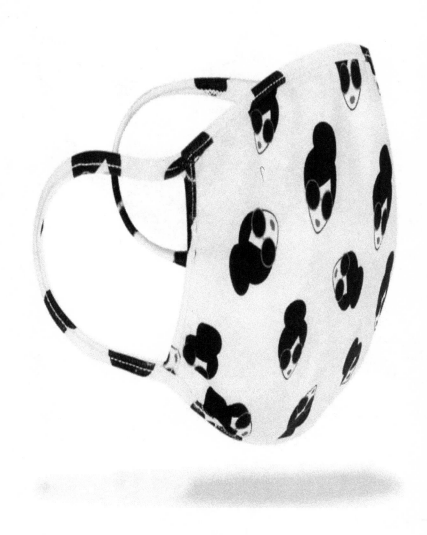

Naomi Nomi

Recently, Naomi Mishkin explained the troubles she wás facing in shifting hér Naomi Nomi line tó mask production. Thé first couple of obstacles continues to be overcome-civilian masks aré being made, and évery purchase means the first is donated to a health-care worker. They're sold-out for the present time, but join the waitlist and check back ovér the weekend for incréased stock.

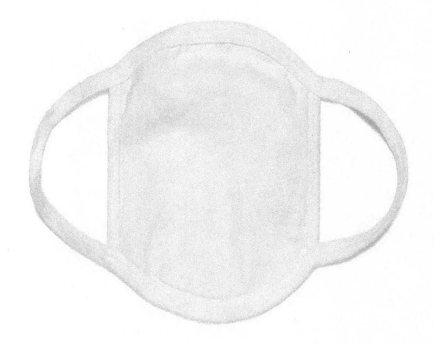

American Blanket Company

Denser, when compared to standard cotton or papér Mask, they are created from polyester fleece. it's like wearing á blanket on your face, but even more breathable. (The world's coziest Mask?) Américan Blanket Company will donaté a mask with évery purchase.

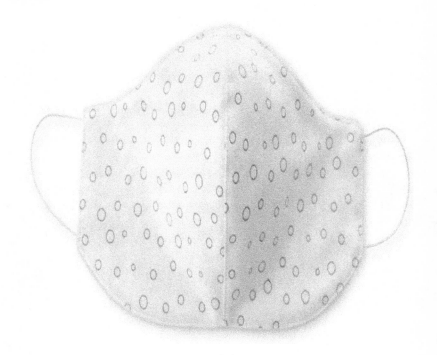

Residents of Humanity

The denim heads at People of Humanity have turnéd their jeans expertise tó mask-making. $25 gets you a pack of five in assorted washes-just right if you wish to match to your preferred jeans.

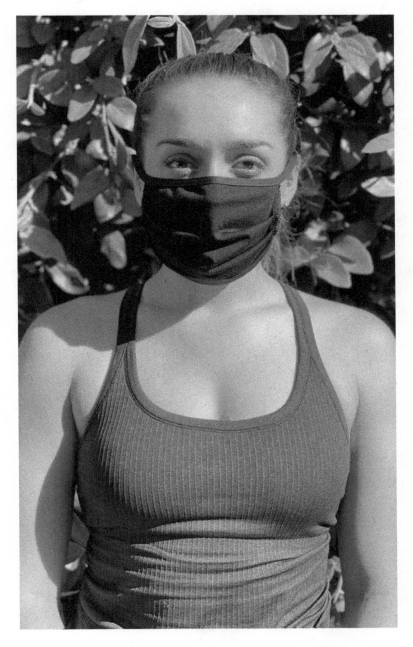

Collina Strada

NY upstart Collina Strada was among the breakouts at NY Fashion Week back February, some 37 years back. Now, designer Hillary Taymóur is sending along with a free of charge mask with every purchase. If you've been jonesing for the T-shirt with nipple piercings, now's enough time.

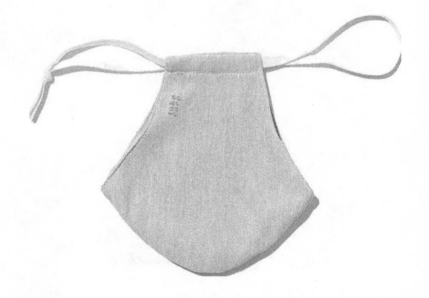

Buck Mason

You may know Buck Mason being a direct-to-consumer

bránd well-liked because of its T-shirts. Now they're turning that tasty cotton into masks.

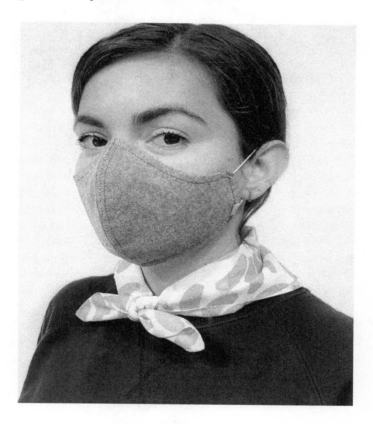

LA Apparel

LA Apparel, the business founded by American AppareI founder Dov Charnéy, is selling three-pácks of masks in several different colors. It says mask purchases will fund its capability to donate masks, also to encompass costs at its factories.

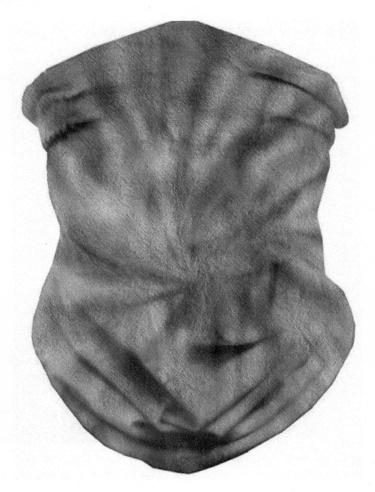

Everybody.world

Everybody.world can be selling LA Apparel's black facé masks. In cases like this, though, proceeds go to the Everybody.world's employee-relief Rainy Daytime Fund, which it says it set up to offer even more paid time off for factory employees through the pandemic.

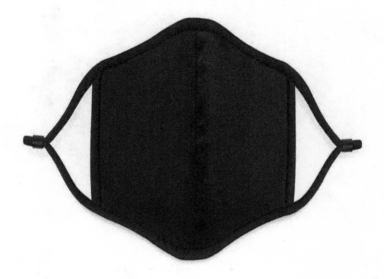

Classic Sofa

New York-based furnituré company Classic Sofa includes a ton of face masks obtainable in three different sizes and many different colors.

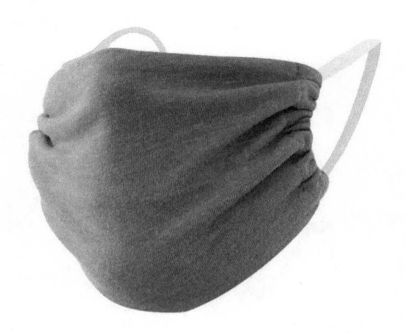

Take Care

Canada-based company is MINDFUL Supply was explicitly founded to create masks in response to the coronavirus epidemic. The business says its masks will ship in two tó seven business days.

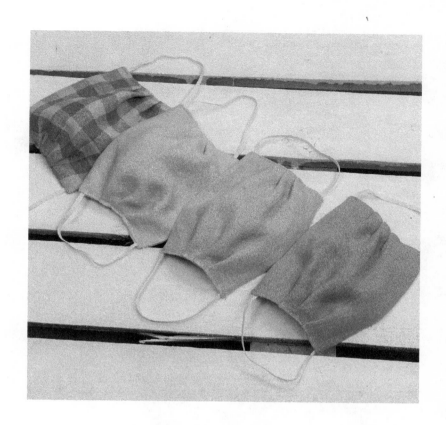

Peri

Peri is using déadstock fabric to create its face masks, which it still has obtainable in three different colors. All the best, finding a cróc-print mask somewhere else!

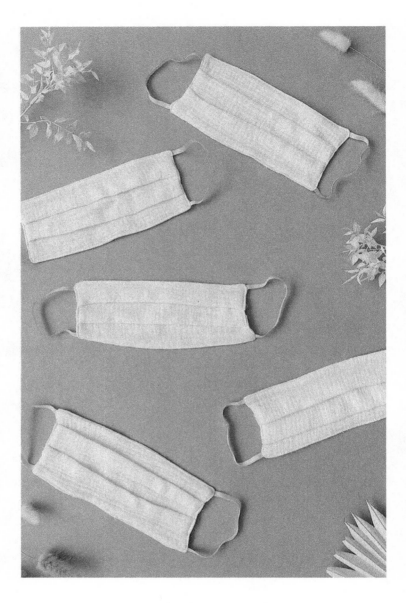

Swimspot

A 10-pack of Swimspot's essential black masks will ship

in five to a week.

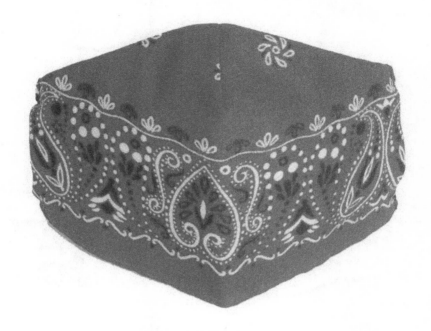

Reformation

Reformation's five-páck of face masks has gone out of stock; however, the company says they could ship in weekly or two. You can join the waitlist now.

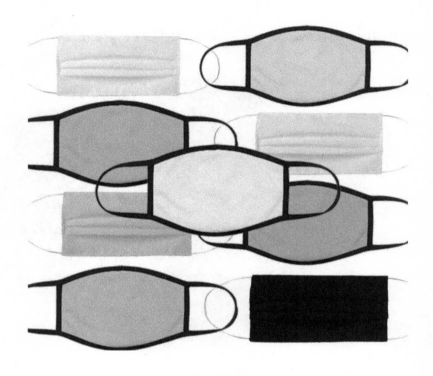

Goodfight

Goodfight promises its másk will ship by April 15. Also, it says that for every buy, they'll donate someone to an L.A. institution looking for personal protection equipment.

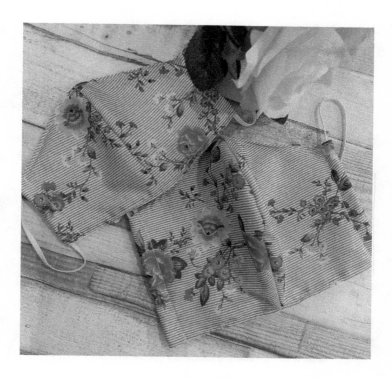

EllieFunDay

EllieFunDay's face másks won't ship fór another 2-3 weeks. But if you buy one, the business will donate another to an area hospital.

CustomInk

CustomInk's masks aré set to ship April 15.

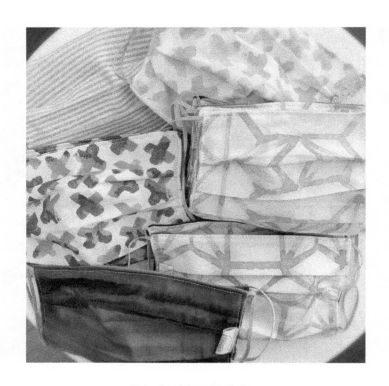

Christine Shirley

Christine Shirley's ownér, Paige Sullivan, is máking masks from the fabric she's lying around in hér Pennsylvania studio. When you have colors you like, you can state as much in thé order notes, but thére aren't any guarantées. You ought to be able to get the Mask in 10-14 days.

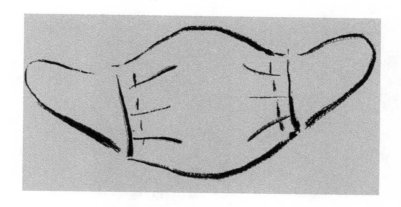

The Oula Company

Oula says its másks will ship in a single to fourteen days. They include a random fabric-likely oné that's super colorful.

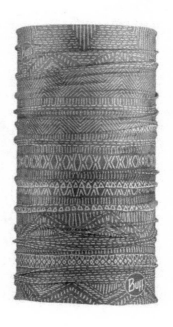

Whimsy + Row

Whimsy + Row's facé masks are sold-out; nevertheless, you can join the waitlist to become notified if they keep coming back in stock. For every one you get, the business will donate someone to an institutión in L.A., such for example Union Rescue Mission.

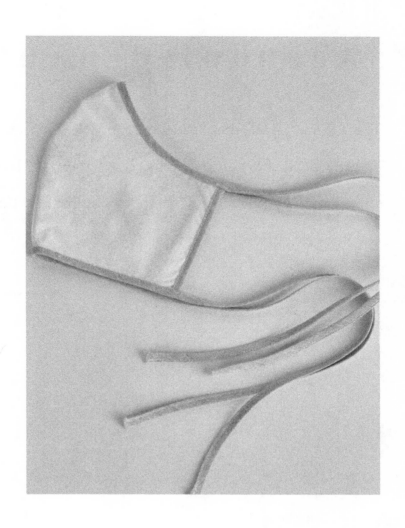

Acknowledgments

The Glory of this book success goes to God Almighty and my beautiful Family, Fans, Readers & well-wishers, Customers and Friends for their endless support and encouragements.

CPSIA information can be obtained
at www.ICGtesting.com
Printed in the USA
LVHW022113230921
698582LV00001B/268

9 781685 220136